RENAL DIET COOKBOOK FOR BEGINNERS 2021

- Eat Healthier and Feel Healthier with Tasty Low Potassium, Low Sodium and Low Phosphorus Recipes -

[Simona Malcom]

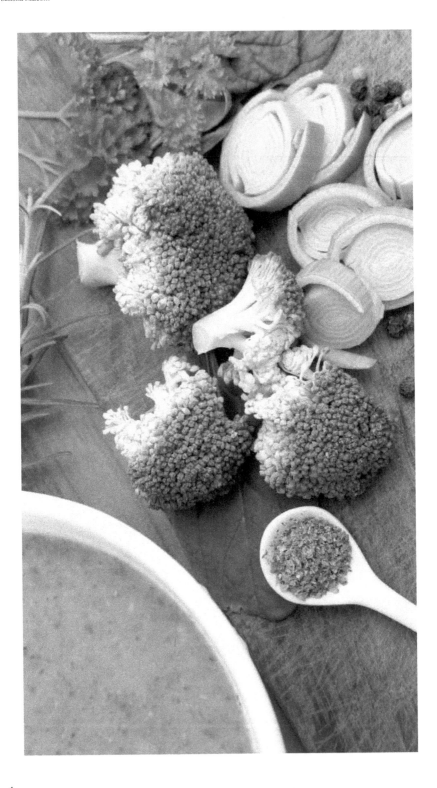

Table Of Contents

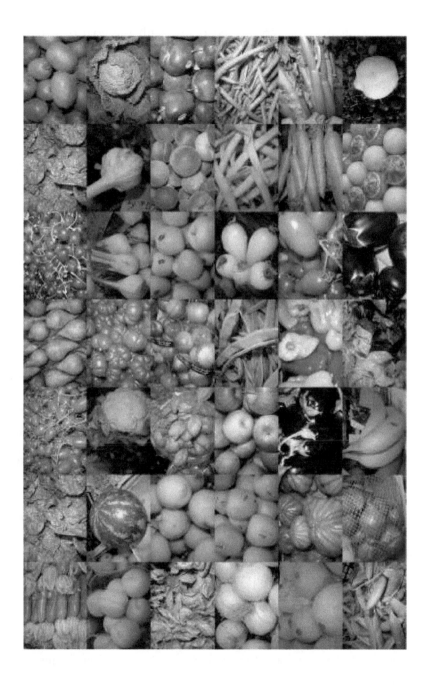

The following Book is reproduced below with the goal of providing information that is as accurate and reliable as possible. Regardless, purchasing this Book can be seen as consent to the fact that both the publisher and the author of this book are in no way experts on the topics discussed within and that any recommendations or suggestions that are made herein are for entertainment purposes only. Professionals should be consulted as needed prior to undertaking any of the action endorsed herein.

This declaration is deemed fair and valid by both the American Bar Association and the Committee of Publishers Association and is legally binding throughout the United States.

Furthermore, the transmission, duplication, or reproduction of any of the following work including specific information will be considered an illegal act irrespective of if it is done electronically or in print. This extends to creating a secondary or tertiary copy of the work or a recorded copy and is only allowed with the express written consent from the Publisher. All additional right reserved.

The information in the following pages is broadly considered a truthful and accurate account of facts and as such, any inattention, use, or misuse of the information in question by the reader will render any resulting actions solely under their purview. There are no scenarios in which the publisher or the original author of this work can be in any fashion deemed liable for any hardship or damages that may befall them after undertaking information described herein.

Additionally, the information in the following pages is intended only for informational purposes and should thus be thought of as universal. As befitting its nature, it is presented without assurance regarding its prolonged validity or interim quality. Trademarks that are mentioned are done without written consent and can in no way be considered an endorsement from the trademark holder.

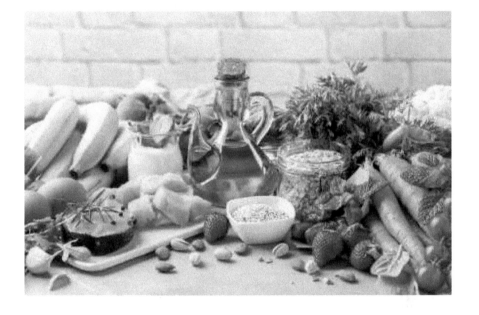

CHAPTER 1: The Renal Diet

The Benefits of Renal diet

If you have been diagnosed with kidney dysfunction, a proper diet is necessary for controlling the amount of toxic waste in the bloodstream. When toxic waste piles up in the system along with increased fluid, chronic inflammation occurs, and we have a much higher chance of developing cardiovascular, bone, metabolic, or other health issues.

Since your kidneys can't fully get rid of the waste on their own, which comes from food and drinks, probably the only natural way to help our system is through this diet.

A renal diet is especially useful during the first stages of kidney dysfunction and leads to the following benefits:

● Prevents excess fluid and waste build-up

● prevents the progression of renal dysfunction stages

● Decreases the likelihood of developing other chronic health problems, e.g., heart disorders

• has a mild antioxidant function in the body, which keeps inflammation and inflammatory responses under control.

The benefits mentioned above are noticeable once the patient follows the diet for at least a month and then continuing it for longer periods to avoid the stage where dialysis is needed. The diet's strictness depends on the current stage of renal/kidney disease if, for example, if you are in the 3rd or 4th stage, you should follow a stricter diet and be attentive to the food, which is allowed or prohibited.

Nutrients You Need

Potassium

Potassium is a naturally occurring mineral found in nearly all foods in varying amounts. Our bodies need an amount of potassium to help with muscle activity as well as electrolyte balance and regulation of blood pressure. However, if potassium is in excess within the system and the kidneys can't expel it (due to renal disease), fluid retention and muscle spasms can occur.

Phosphorus

Phosphorus is a trace mineral found in a wide range of foods and especially dairy, meat, and eggs. It acts synergistically with calcium as well as Vitamin D to promote bone health. However, when there is damage in the kidneys, excess amounts of the mineral cannot be taken out, causing bone weakness.

Calories

When being on a renal diet, it is vital to give yourself the right number of calories to fuel your system. The exact number of calories you should consume daily depends on your age, gender, general health status, and stage of renal disease. In most cases, though, there are no strict limitations in the calorie intake, as long as you take them from proper sources that are low in sodium, potassium, and phosphorus. In general, doctors recommend a daily limit between 1800-2100 calories per day to keep weight within the normal range.

Protein

Protein is an essential nutrient that our systems need to develop and generate new connective tissue, e.g., muscles, even during injuries. Protein also helps stop bleeding and supports the immune system to fight infections. A healthy adult with no kidney disease would usually need 40-65 grams of protein per day.

However, in a renal diet, protein consumption is a tricky subject as too much or too little can cause problems. When metabolized by our systems, protein also creates waste, which is typically processed by the kidneys. However, when kidneys are damaged or underperforming, as in the case of kidney disease, that waste will stay in the system. This is why patients in more advanced CKD stages are advised to limit their protein consumption as well.

Fats

Our systems need fats and particularly good fats as a fuel source and for other metabolic cell functions. A diet high in bad or trans fats can significantly increase the chances of developing heart problems, which often occur with kidney disease. This is why most physicians advise their renal patients to follow a diet that contains a decent amount of good fats and a meager amount of Trans (processed) or saturated fat.

Sodium

Sodium is what our bodies need to regulate fluid and electrolyte balance. It also plays a role in normal cell division in the muscles and nervous system. However, in kidney disease, sodium can quickly spike at higher than normal levels, and the kidneys will be unable to expel it, causing fluid accumulation as a side-effect. Those who also suffer from heart problems as well should limit its consumption as it may raise blood pressure.

Carbohydrates

Carbs act as a major and quick fuel source for the body's cells. When we consume carbs, our systems turn them into glucose and then into energy for "feeding" our body cells. Carbs are generally not restricted in the renal diet. Still, some types of carbs contain dietary fiber as well, which helps regulate normal colon function and protect blood vessels from damage.

Dietary Fiber

Fiber is an important element in our system that cannot be properly digested, but plays a key role in the regulation of our bowel movements and blood cell protection. The fiber in the renal diet is generally encouraged as it helps loosen up the stools, relieve constipation and bloating and protect from colon damage. However, many patients don't get enough amounts of dietary fiber per day, as many of them are high in potassium or phosphorus. Fortunately, there are some good dietary fiber sources for CKD patients that have lower amounts of these minerals compared to others.

Vitamins/Minerals

According to medical research, our systems need at least 13 vitamins and minerals to keep our cells fully active and healthy. However, patients with renal disease are more likely to be depleted by water-soluble vitamins like B-complex and Vitamin C as a result of limited fluid consumption. Therefore, supplementation with these vitamins, along with a renal diet program, should help cover any possible vitamin deficiencies. Supplementation of fat-soluble vitamins like vitamins A, K, and E may be avoided as they can quickly build up in the system and turn toxic.

Fluids

When you are in an advanced stage of renal disease, fluid can quickly build-up and lead to problems. While it is important to keep your system well hydrated, you should avoid minerals like potassium and sodium, which can trigger further fluid build-up and cause a host of other symptoms.

Nutrient You Need to Avoid

Salt or sodium is known for being one of the most important ingredients that the renal diet prohibits its use. This ingredient, although simple, can badly and strongly affect your body, especially the kidneys. Any excess of sodium can't be easily filtered because of the failing condition of the kidneys. A large build-up of sodium can cause catastrophic results on your body. Potassium and Phosphorus are also prohibited for kidney patients depending on the stage of kidney disease.

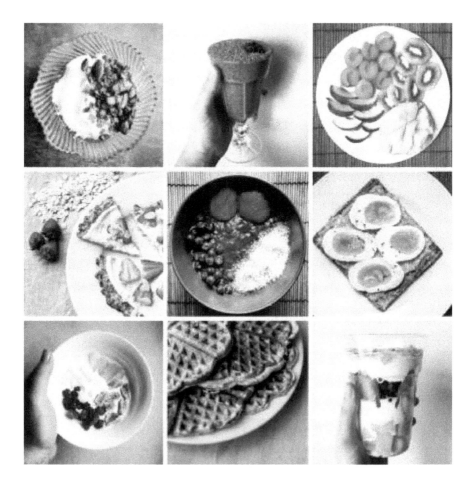

CHAPTER 2: **BREAKFAST**

Mushroom and Tofu Scramble

Prep Time: 20 minutes

Cook Time: 15 minutes

Servings: 3

Ingredients

1 lb firm or extra firm tofu (drained and pressed)

1 ½ cups mushrooms (sliced)

¼ of an onion (diced)

2 tsp dried parsley

½ cup halved cherry tomatoes

1 garlic clove (minced)

½ tsp smoked paprika

½ teaspoon dry mustard

¼ teaspoon tumeric

¼ teaspoon cumin

½ teaspoon salt

⅛ teaspoon pepper

Directions

Drain your tofu and press it for at least 20 minutes.

Wrap your block of tofu in a paper towel and put it on a plate.

Put another plate over the top and weigh it down with bags of dried beans.

In a skillet over medium heat, sauté onion and garlic in 1 tbsp water for a few minutes until soft.

Add the mushrooms and saute until they reduce in volume.

Crumble the tofu into the skillet, add spices and stir to combine.

Cook for a few more minutes to heat through and let the flavors meld.

Take off heat, add tomatoes, stir again to combine.

Serve hot.

Berry Frozen Yogurt

Prep:15 mins

Cook:2 hrs

Servings:4

Ingredients

3 cups plain low-fat yogurt

2 cups blueberries, raspberries and sliced strawberries, mixed

1 cup blueberries, raspberries and sliced strawberries, mixed

1 (1.5 ounce) envelope instant sugar-free vanilla pudding mix

1 tablespoon white sugar

1 tablespoon fresh lemon juice

¾ cup wheat and barley nugget cereal

Directions

Combine the yogurt and pudding mix in a large bowl; beat with an electric mixer until well blended, 1 to 2 minutes. Stir in 2 cups of the mixed berries and the cereal until blended. Pour the yogurt and berry mixture into a 9 inch pie plate. Cover with plastic wrap, and refrigerate 2 hours.

Meanwhile, place the remaining 1 cup of berries in a medium bowl and slightly mash with a fork. Stir in the sugar and lemon juice. Set mixture aside at room temperature.

Nutrition

406 calories

protein 13.5g

carbohydrates 58.7g

fat 14.7g

cholesterol 51.8mg

sodium 708.8mg.

Cinnamon French Toast Strata

Prep:20 mins

Cook:1 hr 30 mins

Additional:13 hrs 10 mins

Servings:15

Ingredients

¾ cup butter, melted

1 teaspoon ground cinnamon

2 (21 ounce) cans apple pie filling

20 slices white bread

6 eggs

1 cup brown sugar

1 ½ cups milk

½ cup maple syrup

1 teaspoon vanilla extract

Directions

Grease a 9x13 inch baking pan. In a small bowl, stir together the melted butter, brown sugar and cinnamon.

2

Spread the sugar mixture into the bottom of the prepared pan. Spread the apple pie filling evenly over the sugar mixture. Layer the bread slices on top of the filling, pressing down as you go. In a medium bowl, beat the eggs with the milk and vanilla. Slowly pour this mixture over the bread, making sure that it is completely absorbed. Cover the pan with aluminum foil and refrigerate overnight.

3

In the morning, preheat oven to 350 degrees F.

4

Place covered pan into the oven and bake at 350 degrees F for 60 to 75 minutes. When done remove from oven and turn on broiler. Remove foil and drizzle maple syrup on top of the egg topping; broil for 2 minutes, or until the syrup begins to caramelize. Remove from the oven and let stand for 10 minutes, then cut into squares. Invert the pan onto a serving tray or baking sheet so the apple filling is on top. Serve hot.

Nutrition

375 calories;

protein 6.1g

carbohydrates 60.5g

fat 12.9g

cholesterol 100.8mg

sodium 370.4mg.

Happy Millet Muffins

Prep:10 mins

Cook:15 mins

Servings:16

Ingredients

2 ¼ cups whole wheat flour

½ cup honey

1 cup buttermilk

⅓ cup millet

 teaspoon baking powder

 teaspoon salt

1 teaspoon baking soda

1 egg, lightly beaten

½ cup vegetable oil

Directions

Preheat oven to 400 degrees F (200 degrees C). Grease 16 muffin cups.

2

In a large bowl, mix the whole wheat flour, millet flour, baking powder, baking soda, and salt. In a separate bowl, mix the buttermilk, egg, vegetable oil, and honey. Stir buttermilk mixture into the flour mixture just until evenly moist. Transfer batter to the prepared muffin cups.

3

Bake 15 minutes in the preheated oven, or until a toothpick inserted in the center of a muffin comes out clean.

Nutrition

176 calories

protein 3.7g

carbohydrates 24.8g

fat 7.7g

cholesterol 12.2mg

sodium 268.4mg.

Berry and Chia Yogurt

Ingredients

1 cup plain nonfat Greek yogurt

1 teaspoon honey

1 Tbsp chia seeds

1 cup fresh or frozen berries

Directions

Combine yogurt and chia seeds in a to-go container.

Mix well.

Add fresh or frozen berries on top of yogurt mixture and lightly drizzle with honey.

Let it sit overnight to allow the flavors to meld and the chia seeds to create a thicker texture.

Nutrition

Calories 300kcal

Total fat 3g

Cholesterol 85 mg

Sodium 85mg

Yufka Pastry Pies

Prep:30 mins

Cook:50 mins

Additional:10 mins

Servings:12

Ingredients

2 cups frozen peas and carrots

1 cup sliced celery

⅔ cup butter

½ teaspoon onion powder

4 (9 inch) unbaked pie crusts

⅔ cup chopped onion

2 cups frozen green beans

1 teaspoon salt

1 teaspoon ground black pepper

½ teaspoon celery seed

½ teaspoon Italian seasoning

1 ¾ cups chicken broth

1 ⅓ cups milk

⅔ cup all-purpose flour

4 cups cubed cooked turkey meat - light and dark meat mixed

Directions

Preheat an oven to 425 degrees F .

2

Place the peas and carrots, green beans, and celery into a saucepan; cover with water, bring to a boil, and simmer over medium-low heat until the celery is tender, about 8 minutes. Drain the vegetables in a colander set in the sink, and set aside.

3

Melt the butter in a saucepan over medium heat, and cook the onion until translucent, about 5 minutes. Stir in 2/3 cup of flour, salt, black pepper, celery seed, onion powder, and Italian seasoning; slowly whisk in the chicken broth and milk until the mixture comes to a simmer and thickens. Remove from heat; stir the cooked vegetables and turkey meat into the filling until well combined.

4

Fit 2 pie crusts into the bottom of 2 9-inch pie dishes. Spoon half the filling into each pie crust, then top each pie with another crust. Pinch and roll the top and bottom crusts together at the edge of each pie to seal, and cut several small slits into the top of the pies with a sharp knife to release steam.

5

Bake in the preheated oven until the crusts are golden brown and the filling is bubbly, 30 to 35 minutes. If the crusts are browning too quickly, cover the pies with aluminum foil after about 15 minutes. Cool for 10 minutes before serving.

Nutrition

539 calories;

protein 20.4g;

carbohydrates 39.5g;

fat 33.2g;

cholesterol 64.7mg;

sodium 650.7mg.

Shrimp Omelet

Prep:30 mins

Cook:25 mins

Servings:3

Ingredients

¼ cup chicken broth

1 (6 ounce) can salad shrimp

1 tablespoon Dijon mustard

2 tablespoons butter

1 (6 ounce) can crab

¼ cup heavy cream

Sauce:

¼ cup heavy cream

1 cup shredded Cheddar cheese

1 dash nutmeg

Salt and pepper to taste

1 teaspoon Dijon mustard

Omelets:

4 eggs, beaten

Salt and pepper to taste

¼ cup heavy cream

Directions

Prepare the filling by stirring Dijon mustard into chicken broth in a saucepan until dissolved. Bring to a simmer over medium-high heat, then add 1/4 cup cream and 2 tablespoons butter. Reduce heat to medium, and simmer until reduced by half, then stir in crab and shrimp; keep warm over low heat.

2

Prepare the sauce by warming 1/4 cup cream, and 1 teaspoon mustard over medium heat. Once hot, whisk in the shredded cheese, then season to taste with nutmeg, salt, and pepper. Keep warm over low heat.

3

Whisk eggs, 1/4 cup cream, salt, and pepper together until smooth. Heat an 8-inch non-stick skillet over medium heat, and lightly oil with cooking spray. Pour 1/4 cup of the egg mixture into hot pan, and swirl to make a thin, even layer of egg. Cook until firmed, then flip and cook for a few seconds more to firm the other side.

4

To prepare omelets, spoon some of the seafood filling into the lower half of each omelet. Roll up into a cylinder. Serve 2 per person bathed with Cheddar sauce.

Nutrition

652 calories;

protein 43.5g;

carbohydrates 4.8g;

fat 50.7g;

cholesterol 536.1mg;

sodium 852.2mg.

Chia Bars

Prep:15 mins

Cook:30 mins

Additional:8 hrs 10 mins

Servings:24

Ingredients

4 cups water, divided

2 teaspoons salt

2 cups chopped almonds

cooking spray

3 cups all-purpose flour

⅔ cup chocolate chips

⅔ cup olive oil

1 pinch salt

⅔ cup chia seeds

½ cup powdered peanut butter (such as PB2®)

1 tablespoon ground cinnamon

2 teaspoons vanilla extract

½ cup honey

Directions

Combine 2 cup water, almonds, and 1 pinch salt together in a bowl; let sit for 8 hours to overnight. Drain and rinse 2 times.

2

Blend drained almonds and 2 cups water together in a blender until smooth, about 2 minutes. Transfer to a large bowl.

3

Preheat oven to 350 degrees F (175 degrees C). Spray an 11x15-inch baking dish with cooking spray.

4

Mix flour, chocolate chips, olive oil, chia seeds, honey, powdered peanut butter, cinnamon, vanilla extract, and 2 teaspoons salt into almond mixture until dough is evenly combined. Transfer dough to the prepared baking dish, leveling dough with a fork or spatula.

5

Bake in the preheated oven until cooked through and lightly browned, 35 - 45 minutes. Allow to cool for 10 minutes before cutting into bars.

Nutrition

248 calories;

protein 5.5g;

carbohydrates 25.8g;

fat 14.8g;

sodium 215.1mg.

Olive Bread

Prep:

20 mins

Cook:

45 mins

Additional:

2 hrs 15 mins

Total:

3 hrs 20 mins

Servings:

24

Yield:

2 loaves

Ingredients

2 ½ cups warm water (110 degrees F/45 degrees C)

2 tablespoons active dry yeast

1 teaspoon molasses

2 tablespoons olive oil

1 tablespoon salt

7 ½ cups bread flour

1 cup kalamata olives, pitted and chopped

2 tablespoons chopped fresh rosemary

1 tablespoon sesame seeds (Optional)

Directions

1

Place water, yeast, and molasses in a mixing bowl; stir to mix. Let stand for a few minutes until mixture is creamy and foamy.

2

Add olive oil and salt; mix. Add flour, about a cup at a time, until dough is too stiff to stir. Add olives and fresh herbs.

3

Turn dough out onto a lightly floured board. Knead, adding flour as needed to keep from being sticky, until smooth and elastic. Place in well oiled bowl, and turn to coat the dough surface with oil. Allow to rise until doubled in bulk, about an hour or so.

4

Punch the dough down, split into two pieces, and form into two round loaves. Place on greased baking sheet . Spray with cold water and sprinkle with sesame seeds if desired. Let loaves rise for 25 to 30 minutes.

5

Bake at 400 degrees F (205 degrees C) for about 45 minutes, or until they are brown and sound hollow when tapped on the bottom.

Nutritions
Per Serving: 186 calories; protein 5.7g; carbohydrates 32.3g; fat 3.6g; sodium 383.9mg.

Toast and Tuna

Prep:

5 mins

Cook:

25 mins

Total:

30 mins

Servings:

3

Yield:

3 servings

Ingredients

1 (10.75 ounce) can condensed cream of mushroom soup
2 hard-cooked eggs, sliced
1 (5 ounce) can tuna, drained
6 slices whole wheat bread

Directions

1

Make cream of mushroom soup according to the directions on the can.

2

Stir in canned tuna and egg slices. Heat thoroughly. Meanwhile, toast bread slices.

3

Spoon tuna mixture over slices of whole wheat toast. Serve.

Nutritions

Per Serving: 317 calories; protein 20.9g; carbohydrates 32g; fat 11.8g; cholesterol 153.9mg; sodium 987.1mg.

CHAPTER 3: LUNCH

Hawaiian Rice

Prep:15 mins

Cook:30 mins

Additional:15 mins

Servings:4

Ingredients

warm water, as needed

3 chicken breasts, or more to taste

water, to cover

1 quart chicken broth

1 small onion, sliced thin

1 (16 ounce) package bean thread vermicelli noodles

3 cloves garlic, chopped

slices fresh ginger, chopped

1 tablespoon patis (Philippine-style fish sauce)

3 bay leaves

salt and ground black pepper to taste

2 cups chopped bok choy

tablespoon soy sauce

Directions

Put bean thread noodles in a large bowl. Pour enough warm water over the noodles to cover by an inch. Soak noodles until softened, about 15 minutes; drain. Cut noodles into shorter lengths as desired.

2

Put chicken breasts in a large pot with enough water to cover by a few inches; bring to a boil and cook chicken until until no longer pink in the center and the juices run clear, 8 to 10 minutes. An instant-read thermometer inserted into the center should read at least 165 degrees F .

3

Remove chicken breasts to a cutting board and shred into strands with 2 forks; return shredded chicken to the pot of boiling water.

4

Pour chicken broth into the pot and reduce heat to medium-high; add onion, garlic, ginger, fish sauce, soy sauce, and bay leaves; season with salt and pepper. Bring liquid again to a boil and add the bean thread noodles; cook at a boil until the noodles are translucent, about 6 minutes.

5

Stir bok choy into the liquid; cook just until the leaves wilt slightly, 1 to 2 minutes.

Nutrition

563 calories; protein 70.6g; carbohydrates 29.4g; fat 20.8g; cholesterol 50.6mg; sodium 1532.9mg.

Avocado - Shrimp Salad

Prep:25 mins

Servings:4

Ingredients

2 avocados - peeled, pitted, and cubed

2 tomatoes, diced

1 pound cooked salad shrimp

1 pinch salt and pepper to taste

2 tablespoons lime juice

1 small sweet onion, chopped

Directions

Stir together avocadoes, tomatoes, onion, and shrimp in a large bowl. Season to taste with salt and pepper. Stir in lime juice. Serve cold.

Nutrition

319 calories; protein 29.1g; carbohydrates 14.9g; fat 17.1g; cholesterol 196.4mg; sodium 203.4mg.

Egg Whites Cups

Prep: 5 Mins

Cook: 5 Mins

Servings: 4

Ingredients

for 6 servings

1 roma tomato, 11 calories

2 cups egg white(480 mL), 250 calories

1 roma tomato, 11 calories

salt, to taste, 0 calories

2 cups spinach(60 g), 14 calories

½ teaspoon pepper, 0 calories

Directions

Preheat the oven to 350°F.

Lightly grease a muffin tin.

Then divide equally the spinach across 6 cups.

Dice the tomato, then fill the cups with the tomato and egg whites.

Season with salt and pepper.

Bake for 15 minutes, or until the whites have set.

Serve hot.

Enjoy!

Nutritions:

Fat 9g

Carbs 1g

Fiber 0g

Sugar 0g

Protein 12g

Sensational Moose Jerky

Prep:1 hr

Cook:12 hrs

Servings:6

Ingredients

3 cups soy sauce

3 pounds rump roast

4 fluid ounces hickory-flavored liquid smoke

3 cups packed brown sugar

Directions

Slice roast into slabs approximately 1/4 inch thick, (Note: you can have this done at the grocery store or butcher). Trim off all of the fat from the edges. Cut the slabs into pencil-like strips (about 1/4 inch wide), and about 4 inches long.

2

In a large bowl, combine the soy sauce, brown sugar and hickory-flavored liquid smoke; blend well. Place all of the meat into the bowl of marinade. Cover and place in refrigerator for at least 30 minutes.

3

Place the meat in a food dehydrator for about 12 to 20 hours, depending how dry you like your jerky. Rotate the trays after 6 hours.

For example: Bottom tray on top, top tray on bottom, second tray from bottom to be second tray from top, and so on.

Nutrition

1129 calories; protein 52.9g; carbohydrates 117.6g; fat 50.5g; cholesterol 138.3mg; sodium 7357.3mg.

Garlic Chicken Balls

Prep: 10 mins

Cook: 10 mins

Servings: 3

Ingredients

500g chicken mince

2 eggs

4 tablespoons butter

2 cups breadcrumbs

3 tablespoons garlic

Cooking oil

1.5 tablespoons parsley

Directions

Melt butter in a small microwave-safe bowl. Mix in crushed garlic and chopped parsley and stir well. Allow your garlic butter mixture to set in refrigerator or freezer until it is firm. It takes 30-60 minutes in the freezer, so you may want to make the day before.

Roll chicken mince into balls, around 2 inches in diameter.

When the garlic butter is set, cut into cubes. Insert one cube of garlic butter into the centre of each mince ball and smooth over with mince, to ensure the butter cube is completely encased.

Whisk eggs in a bowl. Dip chicken balls in egg mixture, then coat generously in breadcrumbs. Repeat with all the chicken balls.

Mujadara (Lentils and Rice with Caramelized Onions)

Prep Time: 25 minutes

Cook Time: 35 minutes

Servings: 4

INGREDIENTS

4 medium cloves garlic, smashed and peeled

2 bay leaves

1 tablespoon ground cumin

1 ¾ teaspoons fine sea salt, divided

5 cups water

1 cup regular brown or green lentils**, picked over for debris, rinsed and drained

⅓ cup extra-virgin olive oil

Freshly ground black pepper

2 medium-to-large yellow onions, halved and thinly sliced

½ cup thinly sliced green onions (from 1 bunch), divided

½ cup chopped fresh cilantro or flat-leaf parsley, divided

1 cup brown* basmati rice (regular, not quick-cooking), rinsed and drained

Plain whole-milk or Greek yogurt, for serving

Spicy sauce, for serving

Directions

In a large Dutch oven or soup pot, combine the garlic, bay leaves, cumin, 1 ½ teaspoons of the salt and about 20 twists of freshly ground black pepper. Add the water and bring the mixture to a boil over medium-high heat.

Once boiling, stir in the rice and reduce the heat to medium. Cover and cook, stirring occasionally and adjusting the heat as necessary to maintain a controlled simmer, for 10 minutes.

Stir in the lentils and let the mixture return to a simmer. Cover again, reduce the heat to medium-low, and cook until the liquid is absorbed and the rice and lentils are tender, about 20 to 23 minutes.

Meanwhile, warm the olive oil in a large (12-inch) skillet over medium-high heat. When it's warm enough that a slice of onion sizzles on contact, add the remaining onions. Stir to combine.

Stir only every 3-4 minutes or so at first, then more often once the onions at the edges of the pan start browning. If the onions are browning before they have softened, dial down the heat to give them more time. Cook until the onions are deeply caramelized and starting to crisp at the edges, about 20 to 30 minutes. In the meantime, line a large plate or cutting board with a couple paper towels.

Using a slotted spoon or fish spatula, transfer the onions to the lined plate and spread them evenly across. Sprinkle the remaining ¼ teaspoon salt over the onions. They'll crisp up as they cool.

When the lentils and rice are done cooking, drain off any excess water (if there is any) and return the mixture to the pot, off the heat. Lay a kitchen towel across the top of the pot to absorb steam, then cover the pot and let it rest for 10 minutes.

Remove the lid, discard the bay leaves, and smash the garlic cloves against the side of the pan with a fork. Add about ¾ths of the green onions and cilantro, reserving the rest for garnish. Gently stir and fluff the rice with a fork. Season to taste with additional salt and pepper, if necessary.

Transfer the rice and lentil mixture to a large serving platter or bowl. Top with the caramelized onions and the remaining green onions and cilantro. Serve hot, warm or at room temperature, with yogurt and spicy sauce (optional) on the side.

Zucchini Sautè

Prep:15 mins

Cook:15 mins

Servings:6

Ingredients

1 tablespoon olive oil

½ red onion, diced

salt and pepper to taste

½ pound fresh mushrooms, sliced

1 teaspoon Italian seasoning

1 tomato, diced

1 clove garlic, minced

4 zucchini, halved and sliced

Directions

Heat oil in a large skillet over medium heat. Saute onion with salt and pepper for 2 minutes. Stir in zucchini and mushrooms. When zucchini begins to soften, add tomatoes, garlic and Italian seasoning. Cook until heated through.

Nutrition

68 calories; protein 2.8g; carbohydrates 9.2g; fat 3.2g; sodium 99.1mg.

Jammin' Jambalaya

Prep:20 mins

Cook:45 mins

Servings:6

Ingredients

2 tablespoons peanut oil, divided

10 ounces andouille sausage, sliced into rounds

1 pound boneless skinless chicken breasts, cut into 1 inch pieces

1 onion, diced

1 tablespoon Cajun seasoning

1 small green bell pepper, diced

3 cloves garlic, minced

1 (16 ounce) can crushed Italian tomatoes

½ teaspoon red pepper flakes

2 stalks celery, diced

½ teaspoon ground black pepper

1 teaspoon salt

2 teaspoons Worcestershire sauce

1 teaspoon file powder

½ teaspoon hot pepper sauce

1 ¼ cups uncooked white rice

2 ½ cups chicken broth

Directions

Heat 1 tablespoon of peanut oil in a large heavy Dutch oven over medium heat. Season the sausage and chicken pieces with Cajun seasoning. Saute sausage until browned. Remove with slotted spoon, and set aside. Add 1 tablespoon peanut oil, and saute chicken pieces until lightly browned on all sides. Remove with a slotted spoon, and set aside.

In the same pot, saute onion, bell pepper, celery and garlic until tender. Stir in crushed tomatoes, and season with red pepper, black pepper, salt, hot pepper sauce, Worcestershire sauce and file powder. Stir in chicken and sausage. Cook for 10 minutes, stirring occasionally.

Stir in the rice and chicken broth. Bring to a boil, reduce heat, and simmer for 20 minutes, or until liquid is absorbed.

Nutrition

465 calories; protein 28.1g; carbohydrates 42.4g; fat 19.8g; cholesterol 73.1mg; sodium 1632.7mg.

Frosted Grapes

Prep:5 mins

Additional:1 hr

Servings:8

Ingredients

2 pounds red seedless grapes

1 (3 ounce) package cherry flavored mix

Directions

Pluck grapes from their stems and rinse in a colander. Pour the gelatin mix onto a plate. Place grapes on the plate one handful at a time and roll around until coated. Transfer to a pretty dish and refrigerate for 1 hour to allow the gelatin to set.

Nutrition

119 calories; protein 1.7g; carbohydrates 29.2g; fat 0.7g; sodium 50mg.

Celery Salad

Prep:

10 mins

Additional:

30 mins

Total:

40 mins

Servings:

2

Yield:

2 servings

Ingredients

¾ cup sliced celery

⅓ cup dried sweet cherries

⅓ cup frozen green peas, thawed

3 tablespoons chopped fresh parsley

1 tablespoon chopped pecans, toasted

1 ½ tablespoons fat-free mayonnaise

1 ½ tablespoons plain low-fat yogurt

1 ½ teaspoons fresh lemon juice

⅛ teaspoon salt

⅛ teaspoon ground black pepper

Directions

1

In a medium bowl, combine the celery, cherries, peas, parsley and pecans. Stir in the mayonnaise, yogurt and lemon juice. Season with salt and pepper. Chill before serving.

Nutritions

Per Serving: 150 calories; protein 4.1g; carbohydrates 26.5g; fat 3g; cholesterol 0.7mg; sodium 304.2mg.

Chicken Tacos

Prep:

15 mins

Cook:

40 mins

Total:

55 mins

Servings:

8

Yield:

8 tacos

Ingredients

¼ cup water

1 (1 ounce) packet taco seasoning mix

2 (8 ounce) cans tomato sauce

2 teaspoons white distilled vinegar

2 teaspoons minced garlic

2 teaspoons ground oregano

1 teaspoon ground cumin

½ teaspoon white sugar

2 tablespoons olive oil

2 pounds skinless, boneless chicken breasts

8 taco shells, warmed

Directions

1

Mix water and taco seasoning in a large bowl. Add tomato sauce, vinegar, garlic, oregano, cumin, and sugar; mix well.

2

Heat oil in a large skillet over medium-high heat. Add chicken and cook until golden brown, about 5 minutes per side. Add tomato sauce mixture and bring to a boil. Reduce heat to medium-low, cover, and simmer until chicken is no longer pink in the center and the juices run clear, about 20 minutes. An instant-read thermometer inserted into the center should read at least 165 degrees F (74 degrees C).

3

Remove chicken breasts from the pan and shred meat with 2 forks when cool enough to handle. Return shredded chicken to the pan with the tomato sauce. Cook and stir until chicken is coated with sauce and sauce reduces a bit, about 5 minutes.

4

Transfer chicken and sauce to a serving bowl and spoon onto taco shells.

Nutritions

Per Serving: 244 calories; protein 24g; carbohydrates 15.7g; fat 9g; cholesterol 58.5mg; sodium 658.8mg.

CHAPTER 4: DINNER

Mussels with Saffron

Prep:35 mins

Cook:35 mins

Servings:6

Ingredients

2 pounds mussels, cleaned and debearded

1 ¼ cups white wine

3 tablespoons margarine

1 tablespoon olive oil

1 onion, chopped

1 ½ cups water

1 clove garlic, crushed

1 leek, bulb only, chopped

1 ½ tablespoons all-purpose flour

6 saffron threads

1 ¼ cups chicken broth

1 tablespoon chopped fresh parsley

½ teaspoon fenugreek seeds, finely crushed

salt and pepper to taste

2 tablespoons whipping cream

Directions

Place saffron threads in a small bowl, and cover with 1 tablespoon boiling water. Set aside.

Scrub mussels clean in several changes of fresh water and pull off beards. Discard any mussels that are cracked or do not close tightly when tapped. Put mussels into a saucepan with wine and water. Cover and cook over high heat, shaking pan frequently, 5-7 minutes or until shells open. Remove mussels, discarding any which remain closed. Strain liquid through a fine sieve and reserve.

Heat butter and oil in a saucepan. Add onion, garlic, leek and fenugreek and cook gently 5 minutes. Stir in flour and cook 1 minute. Add saffron mixture, 2-1/2 cups of reserved cooking liquid and chicken broth. Bring to a boil, cover and simmer gently for 15 minutes.

Meanwhile, keep 8 mussels in shells and remove remaining mussels from shells. Add all mussels to soup and stir in chopped parsley, salt, pepper and cream. Heat through 2-4 minutes. Garnish with parsley sprigs, if desired, and serve hot.

Nutrition

205 calories; protein 9.7g; carbohydrates 9g; fat 10.4g; cholesterol 27mg; sodium 343.1mg.

Broiled Shrimp

Prep:30 mins

Cook:15 mins

Servings:4

Ingredients

2 pounds medium shrimp, peeled and deveined

2 cloves garlic, minced

¼ cup dry white wine

3 green onions, chopped

½ cup butter, melted

Directions

Preheat broiler to 500 degrees .

Stir shrimp together with butter, garlic and wine. Place on a baking sheet and broil for 10 minutes. Sprinkle on scallions and broil for another 2 to 4 minutes, until shrimp are firm. Serve hot.

Nutrition

432 calories; protein 44.8g; carbohydrates 1.3g; fat 26.2g; cholesterol 419.7mg; sodium 672.4mg.

Cilantro Beef

Prep/Total Time: 30 min.

Ingredients

1 beef flank steak (1 pound)

1/2 teaspoon salt

4 teaspoons olive oil, divided

1 medium onion, halved and sliced

1/4 teaspoon pepper

1 jalapeno pepper, seeded and finely chopped

1/2 cup salsa

1/4 cup minced fresh cilantro

2 teaspoons lime juice

1 garlic clove, minced

Dash hot pepper sauce

Optional toppings: salsa, cilantro, shredded lettuce and sour cream

8 flour tortillas (6 inches), warmed

Directions

Sprinkle steak with salt and pepper. In a large skillet, heat 2 teaspoons oil over medium-high heat. Add steak; cook 5-7 minutes on each side or until meat reaches desired doneness (for medium-rare, a thermometer should read 135°; medium, 140°; medium-well, 145°). Remove from pan.

In same skillet, heat remaining oil over medium heat. Add onion; cook and stir 4-5 minutes or until tender. Add jalapeno and garlic; cook 2 minutes longer. Stir in salsa, cilantro, lime juice and pepper sauce; heat through.

Thinly slice steak across the grain; stir into onion mixture. Serve in tortillas; top as desired.

Nutrition

2 tacos (calculated without toppings): 451 calories, 20g fat (7g saturated fat), 54mg cholesterol, 884mg sodium, 38g carbohydrate (3g sugars, 4g fiber), 27g protein.

Wonton Soup

Prep:30 mins

Cook:5 mins

Additional:40 mins

Servings:8

Ingredients

½ pound boneless pork loin, coarsely chopped

1 teaspoon brown sugar

1 tablespoon Chinese rice wine

1 tablespoon light soy sauce

1 teaspoon finely chopped green onion

2 ounces peeled shrimp, finely chopped

24 (3.5 inch square) wonton wrappers

3 cups chicken stock

1 teaspoon chopped fresh ginger root

⅛ cup finely chopped green onion

Directions

In a large bowl, combine pork, shrimp, sugar, wine, soy sauce, 1 teaspoon chopped green onion and ginger. Blend well, and let stand for 25 to 30 minutes.

Place about one teaspoon of the filling at the center of each wonton skin. Moisten all 4 edges of wonton wrapper with water, then pull the top corner down to the bottom, folding the wrapper over the filling to make a triangle. Press edges firmly to make a seal. Bring left and right corners together above the filling. Overlap the tips of these corners, moisten with water and press together. Continue until all wrappers are used.

FOR SOUP: Bring the chicken stock to a rolling boil. Drop wontons in, and cook for 5 minutes. Garnish with chopped green onion, and serve.

Nutrition

145 calories; protein 9.9g; carbohydrates 15.3g; fat 4.2g; cholesterol 32.5mg; sodium 588.8mg

Beef Burritos

Prep:30 mins

Cook:20 mins

Servings:6

Ingredients

6 ounces sliced jalapeno peppers

1 tomato, diced

1 green bell pepper, diced

1 red bell pepper, diced

1 onion, diced

1 ½ tablespoons hot sauce

¼ teaspoon ground cayenne pepper

1 (4 ounce) can chopped green chile peppers

1 pound ground beef

1 (14 ounce) can refried beans

6 (10 inch) flour tortillas

1 (10 ounce) bag shredded lettuce

1 (1 ounce) package burrito seasoning

1 (8 ounce) package shredded sharp Cheddar cheese

1 (8 ounce) container sour cream

Directions

Mix jalapeno peppers, tomato, green chile peppers, green bell pepper, red bell pepper, onion, hot sauce, and cayenne pepper together in a large bowl.

Cook beef in a large skillet over medium-high heat, stirring to break up clumps, about 5 minutes. Drain excess grease. Add jalapeno pepper mixture and burrito seasoning; cook, covered, stirring occasionally, until flavors combine, about 10 minutes.

Pour refried beans into a saucepan over medium-low heat. Cook and stir until heated through, about 5 minutes.

Warm each tortilla in the microwave until soft, 15 to 20 seconds. Spread a layer of refried beans on top. Divide beef mixture among tortillas. Top with lettuce, sour cream, and Cheddar cheese. Fold in opposing edges of each tortilla and roll up into a burrito.

Nutrition

723 calories; protein 34g; carbohydrates 59.9g; fat 38.9g; cholesterol 107.5mg; sodium 2042.5mg.

Carrot Meatballs

Serves 4

Cook: 45 minutes

INGREDIENTS

1 pound ground beef

½ teaspoon black pepper

1 medium yellow onion, minced

2 teaspoons garlic, minced

1 large carrot, grated

1 tablespoon tomato paste

1 teaspoon salt

1 tablespoon dried Italian seasoning

Directions

Preheat oven to 350°F. Lightly grease a baking sheet with cooking spray.

Mix beef, carrot, onion, garlic, Italian seasoning, tomato paste, salt, and pepper, with a fork or with clean hands, until well combined.

Roll into meatballs, roughly one heaping tablespoon in size. Space meatballs apart for even cooking. Bake for 25 minutes.

Remove from oven to rest for 5 minutes before serving.

Oxtail Soup

Prep:20 mins

Cook:12 hrs 10 mins

Additional:1 hr

Servings:8

Ingredients

2 tablespoons butter

1 onion, chopped

½ (750 milliliter) bottle red wine

1 pound beef oxtail, cut into pieces

water to cover

salt and ground black pepper to taste

1 pound potatoes, peeled and cubed

2 ribs celery, chopped

1 cup green beans

2 carrots, chopped

1 (14.5 ounce) can stewed tomatoes

Directions

Heat butter in a large skillet over medium heat. Add oxtail and onion; cook until oxtail is until browned, 6 to 7 minutes per side. Transfer oxtail and onion to a slow cooker.

Pour wine into the skillet and bring to a boil while scraping the browned bits of food off the bottom of the skillet with a wooden spoon. Pour wine mixture into slow cooker; add water to cover.

Set slow cooker to Low; cook soup for 8 hours. Add potatoes, carrots, celery, and green beans; cook soup for 4 hours more.

Cool soup slightly; refrigerate until fat has risen to top and solidified, about 1 hour. Scoop off fat; stir in tomatoes. Reheat soup on stove before serving.

Nutrition

211 calories; protein 11g; carbohydrates 18.7g; fat 6.9g; cholesterol 38.8mg; sodium 241.3mg.

Pad Thai

Prep:40 mins

Cook:20 mins

Servings:6

Ingredients

2 tablespoons butter

1 pound boneless, skinless chicken breast halves, cut into bite-sized pieces

¼ cup vegetable oil

4 eggs

1 (12 ounce) package rice noodles

2 tablespoons fish sauce

3 tablespoons white sugar

1 tablespoon white wine vinegar

2 cups bean sprouts

¼ cup crushed peanuts

⅛ tablespoon crushed red pepper

1 lemon, cut into wedges

3 green onions, chopped

Directions

Soak rice noodles in cold water 35 to 50 minutes, or until soft. Drain, and set aside.

Heat butter in a wok or large heavy skillet. Saute chicken until browned. Remove, and set aside. Heat oil in wok over medium-high heat. Crack eggs into hot oil, and cook until firm. Stir in chicken, and cook for 5 minutes. Add softened noodles, and vinegar, fish sauce, sugar and red pepper. Adjust seasonings to taste. Mix while cooking, until noodles are tender. Add bean sprouts, and mix for 3 minutes.

Nutrition

524 calories; protein 26.4g; carbohydrates 58.5g; fat 20.7g; cholesterol 178.1mg; sodium 593.6mg.

Bamboo Shoots Soup

Prep:10 mins

Cook:23 mins

Additional:15 mins

Servings:2

Ingredients

2 small dried cloud ear mushrooms

1 ½ cups water

4 ounces pork fillet, thinly sliced

2 tablespoons white sugar

2 tablespoons sake (Japanese rice wine)

2 tablespoons soy sauce

4 ounces canned bamboo shoots, drained and chopped

2 tablespoons black rice vinegar

3 eggs

1 ½ teaspoons sesame oil

1 teaspoon chile paste

Directions

Place mushrooms in a small bowl and cover with water. Let soak until softened, about 15 minutes. Drain and cut into bite-size pieces.

Bring 1 1/2 cup water to a boil in a pot. Add pork and bamboo shots. Cook, skimming off any fat that rises to the top, until pork is tender, 7 to 10 minutes.

Mix sugar, sake, soy sauce, black rice vinegar, and chile paste together in a small bowl. Stir into the pot. Reduce heat to low and simmer soup, covered, about 10 minutes.

Stir mushroom pieces into the soup. Crack in eggs and cook, covered, until whites are firm and the yolks have thickened but are not hard, 2 to 3 minutes. Drizzle sesame oil over soup before serving.

Nutrition

323 calories; protein 21.4g; carbohydrates 23.9g; fat 14.7g; cholesterol 305.1mg; sodium 1059.8mg.

Scallops and Brussels Sprouts

YIELD

Makes 4 servings

INGREDIENTS

10 ounces Brussels sprouts, trimmed and halved lengthwise

3 bacon slices (3 ounces), cut crosswise into 1/2-inch pieces

1/4 teaspoon salt

1 cup low-sodium chicken broth

3/4 teaspoon cornstarch

2 teaspoons fresh lemon juice

1/4 cup plus 2 teaspoons water

1 1/2 tablespoons unsalted butter

Pinch of sugar

12 large sea scallops (1 1/4 pounds), tough muscle removed from side of each if necessary

2 teaspoons olive oil

PREPARATION

Blanch Brussels sprouts in a 3- to 4-quart saucepan of boiling salted water , uncovered, 3 minutes, then drain.

Cook bacon in a 10-inch heavy skillet over moderate heat, turning over occasionally, until crisp. Transfer bacon with a slotted spoon to a small bowl and reserve bacon fat in another small bowl.

Add 1/4 cup broth and 1/4 cup water to skillet and bring to a simmer, scraping up any brown bits. Add butter, salt, sugar, a pinch of pepper, and Brussels sprouts and simmer, covered, 4 minutes. Remove lid and cook over moderately high heat, stirring occasionally, until all liquid is evaporated and Brussels sprouts are tender and golden brown, about 8 minutes more. Stir in bacon and remove from heat.

While Brussels sprouts are browning, pat scallops dry and season with salt and pepper. Heat oil with 2 teaspoons bacon fat in a 12-inch heavy skillet over moderately high heat until hot but not smoking, then sear scallops, turning over once, until golden brown and just cooked through, 4 to 6 minutes total. Transfer to a platter as cooked and keep warm, loosely covered with foil.

Pour off and discard any fat from skillet used to cook scallops. Add remaining 3/4 cup broth and simmer, stirring and scraping up any brown bits, 1 minute. Stir cornstarch into remaining 2 teaspoons water in a cup, then stir into sauce along with any scallop juices accumulated on platter. Simmer, stirring, 1 minute, then remove from heat and stir in lemon juice and salt and pepper to taste.

Serve Brussels sprouts topped with scallops and sauce.

Five-Spice Blend

Prep:

10 mins

Cook:

6 mins

Additional:

1 hr

Total:

1 hr 16 mins

Servings:

5

Yield:

5 servings

Ingredients

¼ cup soy sauce

2 tablespoons olive oil

1 tablespoon dry sherry

1 tablespoon orange juice

1 teaspoon minced garlic

1 teaspoon minced fresh ginger root

2 teaspoons Chinese five-spice powder

1 ½ pounds skinless, boneless chicken breast, thinly sliced

Directions

1

Whisk soy sauce, olive oil, sherry, orange juice, garlic, ginger, and Chinese five-spice powder together in a bowl; pour into a resealable plastic bag. Add chicken, coat with the marinade, squeeze bag to remove excess air, and seal the bag. Marinate in the refrigerator at least 1 hour.

2

Preheat grill for medium heat and lightly oil the grate.

3

Remove chicken slices from the marinade; shake to remove excess moisture. Discard remaining marinade.

4

Grill chicken until no longer pink in the center and the juices run clear, about 3 minutes per side.

Nutritions

Per Serving: 234 calories; protein 31.4g; carbohydrates 3.3g; fat 9.8g; cholesterol 83mg; sodium 811.8mg.

Chilaquiles

Prep:

20 mins

Cook:

30 mins

Total:

50 mins

Servings:

8

Yield:

8 servings

Ingredients

1 tablespoon vegetable oil

1 ½ cups thinly sliced red onion

1 jalapeno pepper, seeded and minced

2 (16 ounce) jars salsa verde

1 pound shredded cooked skinless, boneless chicken breast

1 (10 ounce) bag tortilla chips

1 (2.25 ounce) can sliced black olives, drained

¼ cup chopped fresh cilantro

8 eggs

1 dash salt

1 dash ground black pepper

½ cup crumbled cotija cheese

4 radishes, sliced, or to taste

1 avocado, sliced, or to taste

Directions

1

Preheat the oven to 400 degrees F (200 degrees C).

2

Heat oil in a large skillet over medium heat. Add onion and jalapeno; cook, stirring occasionally, until onion begins to brown, about 10 minutes. Transfer to a very large bowl. Add salsa, chicken, chips, olives, and cilantro. Toss to coat, breaking chips slightly. Transfer to a 9x13-inch baking dish.

3

Use the bottom of a custard or measuring cup to make 8 indentations in the chip mixture. Crack 1 egg into each indentation. Sprinkle eggs evenly with salt and black pepper.

4

Bake until eggs are set and tortilla chips are softened and browned at edges, 20 to 25 minutes. Sprinkle with cotija cheese, radishes, and avocado.

Nutritions

Per Serving: 470 calories; protein 27g; carbohydrates 35.2g; fat 24.3g; cholesterol 237.2mg; sodium 838.7mg.

CHAPTER 5: SNACKS AND SIDES RECIPES

Mixes of Snack

Prep:10 mins

Cook:17 mins

Servings:16

Ingredients

Cooking spray

1 cup untoasted walnut halves

½ cup white sugar

1 cup untoasted pecan halves

1 cup unsalted, dry roasted cashews

1 teaspoon salt

½ teaspoon freshly ground black pepper

¼ teaspoon ground cumin

1 cup unsalted, dry roasted almonds

¼ teaspoon cayenne pepper

¼ cup water

1 tablespoon butter

Directions

Preheat oven to 350 degrees F. Line a baking sheet with aluminum foil and lightly coat with cooking spray.

Combine walnut halves, pecan halves, almonds, and cashews in a large bowl. Add salt, black pepper, cumin, and cayenne pepper; toss to coat.

Heat sugar, water, and butter in a small saucepan over medium heat until the butter is melted. Cook for 1 minute and remove from heat. Slowly pour butter mixture over the bowl of nuts and stir to coat. Transfer nuts to the prepared baking sheet and spread into a single layer.

Bake nuts in the preheated oven for 10 minutes. Stir nuts until the warm syrup coats every nut. Spread into a single layer, return to the oven, and bake until nuts are sticky and roasted, about 6 minutes. Allow to cool before serving.

Nutrition

219 calories; protein 4.8g; carbohydrates 12.7g; fat 18.1g; cholesterol 1.9mg; sodium 205.7mg.

Onion Dip

Total:5 mins

Servings:6

Ingredients

¼ cup mayonnaise

1 tablespoon soy sauce

1 tablespoon minced onion

1 ½ teaspoons water, or more as needed

1 tablespoon distilled white vinegar

Directions

Stir the mayonnaise, white vinegar, soy sauce, and water together in a bowl just until combined. Add more water as desired for thinner consistency. Stir in minced onion.

Cover with plastic wrap and refrigerate until cold.

Nutrition

68 calories; protein 0.3g; carbohydrates 0.6g; fat 7.3g; cholesterol 3.5mg; sodium 202.5mg.

Raspberry Vinaigrette Sauce

PREP TIME: 5 mins

TOTAL TIME: 5 mins

SERVINGS: 12 servings

INGREDIENTS

1 1/2 cups raspberries, fresh or frozen

1/4 cup red wine vinegar

1 small shallot, diced (about 2 tbsp)

1/2 cup olive oil

1/4 tsp salt

1 tsp Dijon mustard

pepper, to taste

DIRECTIONS

Add all ingredients to a food processor and blend for 30 seconds.

NUTRITION

CALORIES: 90kcal, CARBOHYDRATES: 2g, FAT: 9g, SATURATE
D
FAT: 1g, SODIUM: 54mg, POTASSIUM: 29mg, FIBER: 1g, VITAMI
N A: 5iu, VITAMIN C: 4.1mg, CALCIUM: 4mg, IRON: 0.2mg

Chimicurri Sauce

Prep: 10 min

Resting: 10 min

Total: 10 min

INGREDIENTS

1/2 cup olive oil

1/2 cup finely chopped parsley

3-4 cloves garlic , finely chopped or minced

2 tablespoons red wine vinegar

3/4 teaspoon dried oregano

1 level teaspoon coarse salt

pepper , to taste (about 1/2 teaspoon)

2 small red chilies , or 1 red chili, deseeded and finely chopped (about 1 tablespoon finely chopped chili)

DIRECTIONS

Mix all ingredients together in a bowl. Allow to sit for 5-10 minutes to release all of the flavours into the oil before using. Ideally, let it sit for more than 2 hours, if time allows.

Chimichurri can be prepared earlier than needed, and refrigerated for 24 hours, if needed.

Use to baste meats (chicken or steaks) while grilling or barbecuing. We don't use it as a marinade, but choose to baste our meats with chimichurri instead. However, you can use it as a marinade if you wish. Also, add a couple of tablespoons over your steak to serve.

Dilled Carrots

Prep:10 mins

Cook:10 mins

Servings:4

Ingredients

3 cups peeled and sliced carrots

2 tablespoons brown sugar

1 ½ tablespoons chopped fresh dill

 tablespoons butter

½ teaspoon black pepper

½ teaspoon salt

Directions

Place carrots in a skillet and pour in just enough water to cover. Bring to a boil over medium heat; simmer until water has evaporated and the carrots are tender. Stir in butter, brown sugar, dill, salt, and pepper.

Nutrition

117 calories; protein 1g; carbohydrates 16.1g; fat 6g; cholesterol 15.3mg; sodium 400.7mg.

Quick Pesto

Prep: 20 mins

Total:20 mins

Servings:24

Ingredients

1 ½ cups baby spinach leaves

½ cup toasted pine nuts

½ cup grated Parmesan cheese

¾ cup fresh basil leaves

¾ teaspoon kosher salt

½ teaspoon freshly ground black pepper

1 tablespoon fresh lemon juice

4 cloves garlic, peeled and quartered

½ cup extra-virgin olive oil

½ teaspoon lemon zest

Directions

Blend the spinach, basil, pine nuts, Parmesan cheese, garlic, salt, pepper, lemon juice, lemon zest, and 2 tablespoons olive oil in a food processor until nearly smooth, scraping the sides of the bowl with a spatula as necessary. Drizzle the remaining olive oil into the mixture while processing until smooth.

Nutrition

67 calories; protein 1.5g; carbohydrates 0.8g; fat 6.6g; cholesterol 1.5mg; sodium 87.2mg

Ants on a Log

Prep:

5 mins

Total:

5 mins

Servings:

1

Yield:

1 log

Ingredients

1 tablespoon peanut butter
1 stalk celery
10 dried cranberries

Directions

1

Spread the peanut butter into the hollow part of the celery. Arrange the cranberries in a line on top of the peanut butter.

Nutritions

Per Serving: 132 calories; protein 4.4g; carbohydrates 12.6g; fat 8.3g; sodium 106.6mg.

Cottage Cheese

Prep:

10 mins

Cook:

10 mins

Total:

20 mins

Servings:

1

Yield:

1 breakfast bowl

Ingredients

2 slices bacon, chopped
2 medium fresh mushrooms, chopped
1 tablespoon minced green onions (including green tops)
salt and ground black pepper to taste
2 eggs, lightly beaten
½ cup cottage cheese

Directions

1

Cook bacon in a small nonstick skillet over medium heat until browned, 4 to 5 minutes. Transfer bacon to a paper towel-lined bowl, reserving bacon grease in a small bowl.

2

Return skillet to medium-high heat and add 1 teaspoon reserved bacon grease. Cook mushrooms and green onions until lightly browned, 3 to

4 minutes. Season with salt and pepper. Transfer to a small bowl and keep warm.

3

Return skillet to medium-high heat and add 1 teaspoon reserved bacon grease. Add eggs and scramble until cooked through, 2 to 3 minutes. Season with salt and pepper. Remove from heat and keep warm.

4

Place cottage cheese into a microwave-safe bowl. Heat on 50% power for 60 to 90 seconds, or until warm, stirring halfway through. Drain any liquid that has been released and transfer cottage cheese into one side of a single-serving bowl. Place scrambled eggs into the other side of the bowl. Top with mushroom mixture and bacon. Serve immediately.

Nutritions

Per Serving: 366 calories; protein 34.5g; carbohydrates 5.7g; fat 22.7g; cholesterol 408.7mg; sodium 1169.3mg.

CHAPTER 6: DESSERTS

Spiced Peaches

Prep:20 mins

Cook:50 mins

Additional:12 hrs

Servings:60

Ingredients

6 cups peeled and chopped fresh peaches

3 cups white sugar

½ teaspoon ground allspice

½ teaspoon ground cinnamon

½ teaspoon ground nutmeg

3 tablespoons lemon juice

Directions

Heat five 12-ounce jars in simmering water until ready for use. Wash lids and rings in warm soapy water.

Mix peaches, sugar, lemon juice, cinnamon, nutmeg, and allspice in a large pot. Bring to a boil; cook, stirring occasionally, until peaches are soft, about 15 minutes. Remove from heat.

Mash peaches with an immersion blender or potato masher to desired size and texture. Return to the heat; continue cooking jam until thickened, about 10 minutes more.

Pack jam into hot jars, filling to within 1/4 inch of the top. Wipe rims with a clean, damp cloth. Top with lids and screw on rings.

Place a rack in the bottom of a large stockpot and fill halfway with water. Bring to a boil and lower in jars using a holder, placing them 2 inches apart. Pour in more boiling water to cover the jars by at least 1 inch. Bring the water to a rolling boil, cover the pot, and process for 10 minutes.

Remove the jars from the stockpot and place onto a cloth-covered or wood surface, several inches apart, until cool, about 12 hours. Press the top of each lid with a finger, ensuring that lid does not move up or down and seal is tight.

Nutrition

43 calories; carbohydrates 10.9g; sodium 0.5mg.

Watermelon Sorbet

Prep:10 mins

Cook:5 mins

Additional:2 hrs 30 mins

Servings:8

Ingredients

1 cup white sugar

3 cups cubed seeded watermelon

¼ cup lemon juice

½ cup water

Directions

Combine sugar, water, and lemon juice in a saucepan over medium heat; cook and stir until sugar is dissolved, about 5 minutes. Remove from heat and refrigerate until cooled, about 30 minutes.

Blend watermelon in a blender or food processor until pureed. Stir pureed watermelon into sugar mixture. Transfer watermelon mixture to an ice cream maker and freeze according to manufacturer's Directions.

Nutrition

116 calories; protein 0.4g; carbohydrates 30g; fat 0.1g; sodium 1.1mg.

Pear Muffins

Prep:15 mins

Cook:20 mins

Additional:25 mins

Servings:12

Ingredients

1 cup whole wheat flour

½ cup all-purpose flour

1 ½ teaspoons baking powder

½ teaspoon salt

½ cup low-fat vanilla yogurt

¾ cup white sugar

½ cup canola oil

1 egg

1 ripe pear - peeled, cored, and diced

½ cup chopped pecans

2 teaspoons vanilla extract

Directions

Preheat oven to 450 degrees F. Grease or line 12 muffin cups with paper liners.

Whisk whole wheat flour, all-purpose flour, sugar, baking powder, and salt together in a bowl. Whisk yogurt, oil, egg, and vanilla extract together in a separate bowl until smooth. Stir yogurt mixture into flour mixture until batter is just mixed; fold in pear and pecans. Spoon batter into the prepared muffin cups.

Place muffin tin in the preheated oven; reduce heat to 350 degrees F. Bake until tops of muffins are browned and a toothpick inserted in the middle comes out clean, 22 to 25 minutes. Cool in the tin for 5 minutes before transferring to a wire rack to cool completely.

Nutrition

240 calories; protein 3.4g; carbohydrates 28.2g; fat 13.4g; cholesterol 16mg; sodium 171.2mg

Vasilopita

Prep:2 hrs 30 mins

Cook:40 mins

Servings: 8

Ingredients

½ cup warm milk

½ cup bread flour

6 cups bread flour

1 (.25 ounce) package active dry yeast

½ cup white sugar

½ teaspoon ground cinnamon

½ teaspoon ground nutmeg

½ teaspoon salt

¾ cup butter, melted

2 cups warm milk

2 tablespoons butter, melted

1 egg, beaten

1 tablespoon water

3 eggs

½ cup chopped almonds

Directions

In a small bowl, stir together 1/2 cup milk, yeast and 1/2 cup flour. Cover and let the sponge rise in a warm place until nearly doubled in size, about 45 minutes.

Place 6 cups flour in a large bowl. Make a well in the center and add the sponge, salt, sugar, cinnamon, nutmeg, 3/4 cup melted butter, 3 eggs and 2 cups milk. Mix thoroughly to make a stiff dough.

Transfer the dough into a greased springform pan. Brush dough with melted butter, cover with greased plastic wrap, and let rise in a warm place until doubled in size, about 60 to 90 minutes.

Preheat oven to 375 degrees F . Beat egg with 1 tablespoon water to make an egg wash.

When dough has risen, insert a clean silver coin into the loaf. Brush dough egg wash and sprinkle with chopped almonds. Bake in preheated oven until deep golden brown, about 40 minutes.

Nutrition

339 calories; protein 7.5g; carbohydrates 18g; fat 27.2g; cholesterol 152.5mg; sodium 355.2mg.

Vanilla Meringue

Prep:20 mins

Cook:1 hr 30 mins

Additional:1 hr 30 mins

Servings:12

Ingredients

2 egg whites

½ cup white sugar

½ vanilla bean

1 tablespoon vanilla extract

⅛ teaspoon cream of tartar

Directions

Preheat the oven to 225 degrees F. Line a large baking sheet with parchment paper.

Place egg whites and cream of tartar into a large bowl; beat using an electric mixer at medium speed until soft peaks form. Increase speed to high and add sugar 1 tablespoon at a time while mixing until stiff peaks form. Scrape seeds from vanilla bean into the bowl and add vanilla extract; beat just until blended.

Spoon batter into a pastry bag and pipe mounds onto the prepared baking sheet.

Bake in the preheated oven until set, about 1 1/2 hours. Turn oven off; let cookies cool in the closed oven for 1 1/2 hours. Remove cookies carefully from paper.

Nutrition

40 calories; protein 0.6g; carbohydrates 9.1g; sodium 9.4mg.

Apple Chia Pudding

Active:10 mins

Total:8 hrs 10 mins

Servings:1

Ingredients

½ cup unsweetened almond milk or other nondairy milk

2 tablespoons chia seeds

¼ teaspoon vanilla extract

1 tablespoon chopped toasted pecans, divided

¼ teaspoon ground cinnamon

½ cup diced apple, divided

2 teaspoons pure maple syrup

Directions

Stir almond milk (or other nondairy milk), chia, maple syrup, vanilla and cinnamon together in a small bowl. Cover and refrigerate for at least 8 hours and up to 3 days.

When ready to serve, stir well. Spoon about half the pudding into a serving glass (or bowl) and top with half the apple and pecans. Add the rest of the pudding and top with the remaining apple and pecans.

Nutrition

233 calories; protein 4.8g; carbohydrates 27.7g; dietary fiber 10.1g; sugars 14.4g; fat 12.7g; saturated fat 1.1g; vitamin a iu 297.7IU; vitamin c 3mg; folate 13.5mcg; calcium 385.9mg; iron 2.1mg; magnesium 84.7mg; potassium 224.2mg; sodium 90.7mg; thiamin 0.2mg; added sugar 8g.

Dutch Apple Pancake

Prep:15 mins

Cook:20 mins

Additional:10 mins

Servings:4

Ingredients

4 eggs

½ cup unbleached all-purpose flour

1 tablespoon sugar

1 pinch salt

½ teaspoon ground nutmeg

1 cup milk

½ teaspoon baking powder

1 teaspoon vanilla extract

½ teaspoon ground nutmeg

¼ cup unsalted butter

2 tablespoons unsalted butter, melted

½ cup white sugar, divided

½ teaspoon ground cinnamon

1 large tart apple - peeled, cored and sliced

Directions

In a large bowl, blend eggs, flour, baking powder, sugar and salt. Gradually mix in milk, stirring constantly. Add vanilla, melted butter and 1/2 teaspoon nutmeg. Let batter stand for 30 minutes or overnight.

Preheat oven to 425 degrees F .

Melt butter in a 10 inch oven proof skillet, brushing butter up on the sides of the pan. In a small bowl, combine 1/4 cup sugar, cinnamon and 1/2 teaspoon nutmeg. Sprinkle mixture over the butter. Line the pan with apple slices. Sprinkle remaining sugar over apples. Place pan over medium-high heat until the mixture bubbles, then gently pour the batter mixture over the apples.

Bake in preheated oven for 15 minutes. Reduce heat to 375 degrees F and bake for 10-12 minutes. Slide pancake onto serving platter and cut into wedges.

Nutrition

456 calories; protein 10.3g; carbohydrates 51.5g; fat 24g; cholesterol 236.6mg; sodium 182.2mg.

Fried Apples

Servings:4

Ingredients

¼ cup vegetable oil

1 pinch salt

¼ cup maple flavored syrup

5 apples - peeled, cored and sliced

Directions

Melt oil or butter in a medium-sized cast iron pan over medium heat. Lay the apple slices in the oil or butter. Cook slowly, turning slices as they start to break down.

When they are soft on both sides, season with a pinch of salt and the syrup.

Nutrition

263 calories; protein 0.4g; carbohydrates 37.5g; fat 14.1g; sodium 13.7mg.

Raspberry Butter

Prep:

10 mins

Additional:

1 hr

Total:

1 hr 10 mins

Servings:

8

Yield:

8 servings

Ingredients

½ cup unsalted butter, at room temperature

¼ cup raspberry preserves

¼ cup fresh raspberries

1 tablespoon confectioners' sugar

Directions

1

Beat butter, raspberry preserves, raspberries, and confectioners' sugar together in a bowl until well combined; refrigerate until set, about 1 hour.

Nutritions

Per Serving: 134 calories; protein 0.2g; carbohydrates 8.3g; fat 11.5g; cholesterol 30.5mg; sodium 1.6mg.

Falafel

Prep:

30 mins

Cook:

20 mins

Additional:

2 days

Total:

2 days

Servings:

6

Yield:

30 falafel

Ingredients

1 cup dried fava beans

water as needed

1 cup dried chickpeas

1 medium onion, coarsely chopped

2 cloves garlic, coarsely chopped

1 bunch flat-leaf parsley, leaves removed

1 pinch cayenne pepper

1 teaspoon ground coriander

¾ teaspoon ground cumin

1 teaspoon baking soda

1 pinch salt and freshly ground black pepper to taste

½ cup vegetable oil for frying, or as needed

Directions

1

Place fava beans in a bowl and cover with plenty of cold water. Soak for 2 days, changing the water daily (in hot weather change the water twice daily).

2

Soak chickpeas on the second day in a separate bowl in plenty of cold water.

3

Drain beans and chickpeas and rinse under cold running water; drain again. Remove the skins from the fava beans and discard them. Do not skip that   or the falafel will not taste good.

4

Combine fava beans, chickpeas, onion, garlic, and parsley leaves in the bowl of a food processor; pulse until pureed, scraping the sides often to ensure everything is evenly processed to a smooth paste. Add cayenne pepper, coriander, cumin, baking soda, salt, and pepper. Transfer to a bowl; cover and let mixture rest for 30 minutes.

5

Line a baking sheet or a large tray with waxed paper.

6

Shape the mixture into 25 to 30 evenly sized patties and place them on the prepared baking sheet, leaving at least 1/2 inch between them. Let rest, uncovered, for 30 minutes.

7

Preheat the oven to 350 degrees F (175 degrees C).

8

Pour oil into the bottom of a large skillet until it just covers the bottom. Heat until oil is hot enough to sizzle a breadcrumb.

9

Carefully lift the falafel from the waxed paper using a spatula. Fry a few falafel at a time and do not overcrowd the skillet. Fry until crisp and brown on the underside, 3 to 5 minutes. Flip, and fry on the other side until browned, another 3 to 5 minutes. Remove from skillet and transfer to a baking sheet. Place the finished falafel in the preheated oven to keep warm while you fry the rest, adding more oil to the pan as needed.

CHAPTER 7: SMOOTHIES AND DRINKS

Caramel Latte

Ingredients

3 fluid ounces brewed espresso

1 tablespoon caramel sauce

2 tablespoons whipped cream

¾ cup milk

½ cups ice cubes

2 tablespoons white sugar

Directions

Place the espresso, caramel sauce, and sugar into a blender pitcher. Blend on high until the caramel and sugar dissolve into the espresso. Pour in the milk and add the ice; continue blending until smooth and frothy. Top with whipped cream to serve.

Nutrition

293 calories; protein 6.8g; carbohydrates 47.5g; fat 9.3g; cholesterol 35.4mg; sodium 164.1mg.

Nectarin Juice

Prep:5 mins

Cook:0 mins

Total:5 mins

Ingredients

2 Nectarines

1-2 tablespoons of your favorite seeds or nuts such

as Pumpkin, Walnut, Sesame or Almond

For a wonderful smoothie add 1-2 cups of Oat, Rice, Almond or cow's

milk

3-4 leaves of your favorite green such as Kale, Spinach or my

favorite, Wheatgrass

2 Carrots

Directions

Gather the ingredients.

Blend.

Note that there are no added sweeteners even in this smoothie recipe.

This is because the recipe is delicious without added sugar.

Grape Drink

Prep Time5 mins

Cook Time20 mins

Ingredients

For Grape Juice

300 grams grapes seedless

1/2 lemon

400 ml water

5 to 6 Ice Cubes

1/3 cup sugar

For Grape Soda

250 ml soda water

lemon wedge

½ sprig mint leaves

Directions

Making Grape Juice

Pour water into a saucepan.

Add seedless grapes and bring to a boil.

When the water starts to boil. Add sugar and mix well.

Add lemon juice to prevent the sugar from caramelizing.

Boil for 15 to 20 minutes and turn off the flame.

Leave until it cools down to room temperature.

Later make them into juice and transfer it into a clean & dry jar, store in the refrigerator.

Making Grape Soda

Take Ice Cubes into a glass.

Add ¼ cup Grape Juice.

Pour soda water.put a lemon wedge and a mint sprig and serve chilled.

Almond Milk

Prep:10 mins

Cook:3 mins

Servings:4

Ingredients

4 cups water, divided

¼ cup raw unsalted almonds

1 tablespoon tapioca flour

1 teaspoon soy lecithin

1 dash vanilla extract

Directions

Combine 1 cup water and tapioca flour in a microwave-safe cup; heat in microwave until boiling, about 4 minutes.

Combine tapioca mixture, remaining 3 cups water, almonds, soy lecithin, and vanilla extract in a high-powered blender; blend on high until smooth.

Strain mixture through cheese cloth layers into a container. Keep refrigerated.

Nutrition

68 calories; protein 1.9g; carbohydrates 3.5g; fat 5.6g; sodium 7.3mg

Conclusion

Kidney disease is now ranked as the 18th deadliest disease in the world. In the United States alone, it is estimated that more than 600,000 Americans have kidney failure.

These statistics are concerning, so it is essential that you take proper care of your kidneys, starting with a kidney-friendly diet.

In this e-book, you will learn that management creates healthy, tasty, and kidney-friendly dishes.

These recipes are ideal whether you have been diagnosed with a kidney problem or want to avoid it.

When it comes to your well-being and health, it's a good idea to visit your doctor as often as possible to make sure you don't experience problems that you may not have. The kidneys are your body's channel for toxins (like the liver), cleaning the blood of distant substances and toxins that are flushed out by things like food preservatives and other toxins.

Where you eat fluffy and fill your body with toxins, whether from food, beverages (for example, drink or alcohol) or even the air you breathe (free radicals are in the sun and move through your skin, through dirty air), and many food sources contain them). Your body will generally convert a lot of things that appear to be benign until your body organs convert them to things like formaldehyde due to the synthetic response and metamorphic phase.

An example is a large part of these dietary sugars that are used in sodas. For example, aspartame is converted to formaldehyde in the body. These toxins must be removed, or they can cause disease, kidney failure, malignancy, and various other painful problems.

This is not a situation that happens without any predictions; it is a dynamic problem and in the sense that it can be found as soon as it can be treated, change the diet, and it is possible what is causing the problem. You may still have partial kidney failure, as a rule. It takes a little time (or a completely terrible diet for a short period of time) to reach complete kidney failure. You would rather not have total kidney failure as this will require standard dialysis treatments to save your life.

Dialysis treatments explicitly cleanse the blood of wastes and toxins in the blood using a machine, taking into account the fact that your body can no longer be held responsible. Without treatment, you could die a very painful death. Kidney failure can be a consequence of long-term diabetes, hypertension, and unreliable diet, and can be the result of other health problems.

A kidney diet is related to the orientation of protein and phosphorus intake in your eating routine. It is also important to limit your sodium intake. By controlling these two variables, you can control the vast majority of toxins/wastes produced by your body and thus allow your kidney to function at 100%. If you do this early enough and really moderate your diets with extreme caution, you could prevent complete kidney failure. If you receive it early, you can fix it completely.

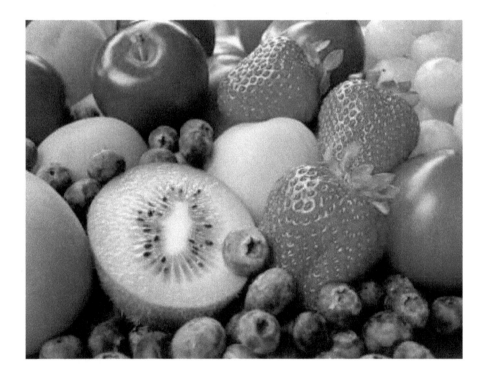

CPSIA information can be obtained
at www.ICGtesting.com
Printed in the USA
LVHW050543160621
690357LV00008B/1243